THE PATH TO PAIN-FREE CHILDBIRTH

A Comprehensive Guide to Natural Techniques, Holistic Practices, and Mind-Body Approaches for an Empowering and Comfortable Birth Experience

By

Sharon G. Brown

TABLE OF CONTENT

Greetings, expectant mothers! Childbirth can be a positive and empowering experience, free from unnecessary pain and challenges. The idea of pain-free childbirth is based on the notion that through proper preparation, mindset, and techniques, you can have a serene and comfortable birth experience.

Choosing a pain-free approach to childbirth provides a wide range of physical, emotional, and psychological advantages. Discover the multitude of benefits that come with pain-free birthing methods, including reduced stress and anxiety, faster recovery times, and a deeper connection with your baby. This book explores the many positive outcomes that can be achieved through these engaging techniques. We will also explore how a pain-free birth can contribute to a more empowering and fulfilling birth experience.

This book aims to provide expectant mothers with a complete guide to achieving a pain-free childbirth experience. Whether you're just starting out or already have some experience, you'll discover valuable insights and practical tips within these pages. Each chapter builds on the previous one, providing a step-by-step approach to preparing for and achieving a pain-free birth. This indispensable guide promises to be a valuable resource, an uplifting source of ideas, and a trusted companion to help you achieve a peaceful and joyful delivery.

CHAPTER ONE

Preparing for a Birth with Minimal Discomfort

The Mind-Body Connection

The mind-body connection is essential for achieving a pain-free childbirth. This concept highlights the interconnectedness of the mind and body, suggesting that by cultivating a positive mental state, one can impact their physical experience of birth. Gaining an understanding of how stress and fear can intensify pain, and how relaxation and confidence can alleviate it, is crucial to this approach. Various techniques, including meditation, visualization, and mindful breathing, will be explored to assist in harnessing the potential of the mind-body connection. Having a positive mindset is crucial when it comes to preparing for a pain-free birth. Developing a positive mindset, self-assurance, and a composed attitude can greatly influence your childbirth experience. This section will offer practical strategies to help individuals address and manage common fears and anxieties associated with childbirth. These techniques include affirmations, journaling, and cognitive-behavioral methods. By adopting a rational and logical mindset, you can approach labor with a sense of confidence and preparedness.

A carefully considered birth plan is also crucial part of preparing for a comfortable childbirth. This plan provides a comprehensive outline for your birth experience, outlining your preferences and ensuring that all parties involved are well-informed of your desires. This section will provide you with a step-by-step guide on how to create a birth plan. It will cover important factors such as natural pain relief methods, your preferred birth environment, and effective communication with your healthcare team. We will provide you with examples of birth plans and templates to assist you in customizing your own.

Prenatal Care and Practices

- **Eating Well During Pregnancy**

Having a well-balanced diet during pregnancy is crucial for the well-being of both the mother and the growing baby. A well-rounded and nourishing diet is crucial for promoting fetal development, ensuring the mother's health, and getting the body ready for childbirth. These are the dietary recommendations, and practical tips for maintaining a healthy diet during pregnancy.

Folic Acid (Folate):

Crucial in the prevention of neural tube defects and in promoting the growth of the fetal brain and spinal cord.

Here are some sources of this essential nutrient: leafy green vegetables like spinach and kale, legumes such as lentils and beans, citrus fruits, nuts, and fortified cereals.

Iron:

Vital for the synthesis of hemoglobin, which facilitates the transportation of oxygen in the bloodstream. Iron requirements are heightened during pregnancy in order to provide adequate support for the developing baby and placenta.

Recommended sources of nutrition include lean meats, poultry, fish, fortified cereals, beans, spinach, and iron supplements if advised by your healthcare provider.

Calcium:

Crucial for the growth and strength of the baby's bones and teeth, while also playing a key role in preserving the mother's bone health.

Sources: Dairy products like milk, cheese, and yogurt, fortified plant-based milk such as almond and soy, leafy greens, and calcium-fortified foods.

Protein:

Facilitates the development of fetal tissues, including the brain, and aids in preserving the mother's muscle mass.

Here are some sources of protein: lean meats, poultry, fish, eggs, dairy products, legumes, nuts, and seeds.

Omega-3 Fatty Acids:

Crucial for the development of the fetal brain and eyes.

Here are some sources of this nutrients that are beneficial for brain health: fatty fish like salmon and sardines, flaxseeds, chia seeds, walnuts, and fish oil supplements.

Vitamin D:

Facilitates the absorption of calcium and enhances immune system functionality.

Sources: Sunlight exposure, fatty fish, fortified milk, and egg yolks.

Vitamin C:

Boosts the immune system, improves iron absorption, and fosters the health of skin and tissues.

Some sources of essential nutrients include citrus fruits like oranges and grapefruits, strawberries, bell peppers, and broccoli.

Fiber:

Assists in mitigating constipation, a prevalent concern during pregnancy.

Sources: Whole grains, fruits, vegetables, legumes, and nuts.

Guidelines for a Healthy Diet

Enjoy a Diverse Range of Culinary Delights:

Incorporate a diverse selection of foods to guarantee a well-rounded intake of nutrients. Emphasize the importance of consuming whole foods like fruits, vegetables, whole grains, lean proteins, and healthy fats.

Stay properly hydrated:

It is important to consume an adequate amount of water in order to maintain proper hydration. This is beneficial for supporting optimal blood volume and amniotic fluid levels. Strive to consume a minimum of 8-10 glasses of water daily.

Regular, frequent meals:

Consuming smaller, more frequent meals can be beneficial in alleviating the discomfort of nausea and heartburn, both of which are frequently experienced during pregnancy. This also aids in sustaining consistent energy levels.

Reduce processed foods

It is advisable to reduce the consumption of processed and sugary foods as they provide minimal nutritional value and can contribute to weight gain and various health issues.

Steer clear of certain food items:

Avoid consuming foods that have the potential to cause foodborne illnesses, like dairy products that haven't been pasteurized, meats that are raw or not fully cooked, certain types of fish that contain high levels of mercury (such as shark, swordfish, and king mackerel), and deli meats that haven't been heated properly.

Prenatal Vitamins:

Follow the guidance of your healthcare provider and make sure to include prenatal vitamins in your routine. These vitamins are essential for providing your body with the necessary nutrients such as folic acid, iron, and calcium.

Useful Suggestions Meal Planning

It is wise to carefully plan your meals and snacks in advance to guarantee that you have a variety of nutritious choices at your disposal. Engaging in meal preparation and planning ahead can be a valuable time-saving strategy that also helps alleviate stress.

Smart Snacking:

Make sure to have a selection of healthy snacks readily available, like yogurt, nuts, fresh fruit, and whole-grain crackers, to sustain your energy levels throughout the day.

Giving into Your Body:

Be mindful of your body's hunger and fullness signals, and nourish yourself when you feel the need. Shift your perspective away from the notion of "eating for two" and instead prioritize the quality of the food you consume.

Controlling Desires and Dislikes:

It is a common occurrence to have food cravings and aversions while pregnant. Strive to discover nutritious alternatives for cravings and experiment with various foods if you develop dislikes for certain ones.

Consider consulting with a knowledgeable expert:

Seek guidance from a registered dietitian or your healthcare provider to receive tailored nutrition advice and address any particular dietary concerns or conditions, such as gestational diabetes.

By adhering to these nutritional guidelines and prioritizing a well-rounded diet, you can promote your baby's growth and improve your own health during pregnancy. A well-balanced diet forms the basis for a comfortable and optimistic childbirth experience.

CHAPTER TWO

Physical Conditioning and Exercise

Pregnancy-related physical activity is crucial for preserving general health, getting the body ready for labor, and encouraging a speedier postpartum recovery.

Exercise Advantages for Pregnancy:

Better Physical Health

- Improves flexibility, muscle strength, and cardiovascular health.
- Lowers the chance of preeclampsia, gestational diabetes, and excessive weight gain.
- Helps with common pregnant discomforts include constipation, edema, and back pain.

Improved Mental Well-Being:

- Energizes and elevates mood.
- Lowers anxiety, stress, and depressive symptoms.
- Enhances the quality of sleep.

Simpler Delivery and Labor:

- Improves endurance and stamina for work.
- Builds up the muscles needed for birthing.
- Enhances coping mechanisms and pain threshold.

Quicker Postpartum Recuperation:

- Speeds up the process of returning to pre-pregnancy fitness levels.
- Lowers the possibility of postpartum depression.
- Fosters confidence and general well-being.

Safe and Effective Exercise

➢ **Walking**

A simple, low-impact workout that fits well into regular schedules. It aids in maintaining a healthy weight and strengthening cardiovascular health.

➢ **Swimming:**

It reduces joint stress while offering a full-body workout. Helps increase circulation and reduce edema.

➢ **Yoga for expectant mothers:**

Emphasizes relaxation, strength, and flexibility. It improves breathing methods and encourages serenity of mind.

➢ **Kegel exercises for the pelvic floor:**

Strengthens the muscles of the pelvic floor, which support the bowels, bladder, and uterus. Supports the body throughout birth and aids in the prevention of urine incontinence.

Strengthening Exercise

Strengthening exercise incorporates resistance bands or small weights to keep muscles toned. It concentrates on the main muscle groups, especially the arms, back, and legs.

Stretching:

- Eases tense muscles and increases flexibility.
- Improves range of motion and keeps muscles from cramping.

Advice for Expectant Mothers

See Your Healthcare Provider:

Get your doctor's approval before beginning any fitness program to make sure it is safe for your particular condition.

Pay Attention to Your Body:

Observe how your body feels and refrain from exerting too much energy. As your pregnancy goes on, adjust the workouts and take breaks as needed.

Maintain Hydration:

To stay hydrated, sip in lots of water prior to, during, and following physical activity.

Put on Cozy Clothes:

Choose supportive footwear and clothes that are elastic and breathable.

Warm-Up and Cool Down:

Warming up at the start of each activity helps your muscles become ready, and cooling down at the conclusion helps your heart rate go down gradually.

Steer clear of certain activities:

After the first trimester, stay away from contact activities, high-impact sports, and workouts that need you to lie flat on your back.

Techniques for Stress Management

For the mother's and the unborn child's health and wellbeing, stress management is essential throughout pregnancy. Having good stress management techniques is crucial since high levels of stress can have a detrimental influence on pregnancy outcomes.

Mindfulness Meditation

Engage in mindfulness meditation to maintain attention and awareness. Deep breathing, body scanning, and guided visualization are some of the techniques used to ease anxiety and encourage relaxation.

Breathing Techniques:

Practice deep breathing techniques to help your nervous system relax. Try taking a deep breath through your nose, holding it for a short while, and then gently letting it out through your mouth.

Progressive Relaxation of the Muscles:

Systematically tension, then release, various bodily muscular groups. This encourages general relaxation and relieves physical strain.

Yoga for expectant mothers:

Use prenatal yoga to incorporate breathing techniques, mindfulness, and physical activity. Yoga promotes mental clarity, flexibility, and stress reduction.

Writing a Journal:

Put your ideas, emotions, and experiences down in writing. Maintaining a journal can be a therapeutic means of managing stress and processing emotions.

Choosing a Healthier Lifestyle:

Eat a healthy, balanced diet, exercise frequently, and get enough sleep. Stress is decreased and general well-being is enhanced by a healthy lifestyle.

Social Assistance:

Communicate with loved ones, friends, and support networks. Feelings of stress and loneliness can be considerably reduced by talking about experiences and getting support from others.

Aromatherapy:

Employ calming essential oils, such chamomile or lavender, to create a relaxing atmosphere. Stress relief and relaxation are two benefits of aromatherapy.

Effective Time Management:

Set attainable objectives and prioritize your work. Assign tasks to others and take pauses to prevent burnout.

Expert Assistance:

If stress becomes too much for you to handle, get expert assistance in mental health. Counselors and therapists can offer coping mechanisms and emotional support.

Helpful Tips to Managing Pregnancy Stress

Establish a Calm Routine:

Every day, set aside some time for soothing pursuits like deep breathing, meditation, or a warm bath.

Establish Boundaries:

Learn to decline extra responsibilities that could put you under unnecessary stress. Put your well-being first and concentrate on self-care.

Exercise Gratitude:

Maintain a thankfulness diary to help you remember the good things in your life. Reducing stress and changing your perspective are two benefits of thankfulness.

Take Part in Hobbies:

Whether it's reading, crafts, or just spending time in nature, do what you enjoy. Taking part in hobbies can make you happy and calm.

Remain educated, but not overwhelmed:

Learn as much as you can about getting pregnant and giving birth, but don't learn too much at once. Select trustworthy sources and restrict your exposure to unfavorable news.

You may improve your physical and emotional health throughout pregnancy by including these stress-reduction and exercise routines into your daily schedule. Maintaining an active lifestyle and practicing effective stress management will set you up for a more comfortable and seamless delivery.

CHAPTER THREE

Natural Pain Relief Techniques

Breathing Techniques and Relaxation

Natural pain management during childbirth relies heavily on breathing and relaxation techniques. These approaches help to manage labor pain, reduce anxiety, and foster a sense of calm and control.

Deep Breathing:

Description: Take slow, deep breaths to boost oxygen intake and induce calm.

How to Practice:

Inhale deeply through your nose, letting your abdomen expand.

Hold your breath for a count of four.

Exhale softly through your lips, releasing any tension.

Benefits include decreased stress hormones, lower blood pressure, and a rhythm to focus on during contractions.

Patterned Breathing:

Description: A rhythmic breathing method that is commonly utilized during labor.

To practice, breathe in through your nose and count to four.

Breathe out through your mouth for a count of four.

Adjust the counts to get a comfortable rhythm.

Benefits include improved focus, reduced pain perception, and a sensation of control.

Breath Awareness:

Description: Stay present by focusing on the natural rhythm of your breath.

Practice by sitting or lying down comfortably.

Close your eyes and pay attention to your breathing.

Take note of the inhale and exhale without attempting to adjust them.

Benefits: Increases mindfulness, lowers anxiety, and promotes a tranquil condition.

Progressive relaxation:

Description: Each muscle group is systematically tensed and subsequently relaxed.

To practice, start with your toes and work your way up to your head.

Tense each muscle group for a few seconds before releasing.

Concentrate on the difference between stress and relaxation.

Benefits: Reduces physical stress, promotes relaxation, and can be utilized in between contractions.

Hypnobirthing Methods

Hypnobirthing is a childbirth practice that employs self-hypnosis techniques to induce a calm and relaxed condition, hence minimizing pain and fear during labor. It combines deep relaxation, visualization, and positive affirmations.

Self-Hypnosis:

Description: A condition of focused calm in which you are particularly open to suggestions.

How to Practice:

Find a quiet, comfortable spot to sit or lie down.

Use a calming voice or tape to help you relax.

Concentrate on positive affirmations and thoughts of a peaceful, gentle birth.

Benefits: Lowers fear and anxiety, reduces pain perception, and fosters a sense of control and empowerment.

Visualization:

Description: Visualizing a tranquil and happy birth experience.

Practice: Close your eyes and visualize your perfect delivery setting.

Visualize your ideal environment, noises, and sensations.

Repeat these visualizations on a daily basis to help you maintain a good mindset.

Benefits: Promotes relaxation, confidence, and a pleasant relationship with birthing.

Positive affirmations:

Repeating encouraging statements to maintain a calm and confident attitude.

How to Practice:

Make a list of affirmations like, "My body knows how to birth my baby" or "I am calm and in control."

Repeat these affirmations daily, particularly during relaxation or self-hypnosis sessions.

Use them during labor to stay focused and optimistic.

Benefits: Increases self-confidence, lowers negative thinking, and improves mental resilience.

Visualization and Meditation Practices

Visualization and meditation are effective methods for pain management and relaxation during labor. These techniques serve to focus the mind, minimize stress, and build a healthy mental environment for labor.

➤ **Guided Imagery:**

Description: A guide (recorded or person) leads you through a sequence of relaxing mental imagery.

How to Practice:

Locate a comfortable position and close your eyes.

Listen to a guided imagery recording that depicts a tranquil setting, such as a beach or garden.

Use all of your senses to make the imagery vivid and engaging.

Benefits: Promotes deep relaxation, distracts from discomfort, and fosters a happy mental environment.

> **Body Scan Meditation:**

Description: A type of mindfulness meditation in which you mentally scan your body for tension and release it.

To practice, lie down comfortably and close your eyes.

Begin with your toes and mentally scan up to your head, noting any points of tightness.

Breathe into each tense place, imagining the tension fading away.

Benefits: Increases body awareness, relieves stress, and promotes relaxation.

➢ **Affirmation Meditation:**

Combining meditation and positive affirmations to achieve a focused and positive mental state.

How to Practice:

Sit comfortably and close your eyes.

Choose a positive affirmation and say it silently or aloud.

Allow the affirmation's meaning to permeate your thoughts.

Benefits: Strengthens positive thoughts, lowers stress, and fosters a calm and confident attitude.

Breath-focused meditation:

Using the breath as a focal point for meditation can help foster calm and attention.

How to Practice:

Sit or lie in a comfortable position.

Close your eyes and pay attention to your breathing.

Take note of the sensation of the breath entering and exiting your body.

If your thoughts wander, gently bring them back to the breath.

Benefits: Increases awareness, decreases tension, and promotes a state of calm and focus.

By including these practices throughout your labor preparation, you can ensure a more comfortable and empowering birth experience. Each approach provides distinct advantages and may be adapted to your preferences and requirements. Practice consistently to gain confidence and familiarity, making these strategies more accessible during birth.

CHAPTER FOUR

The Importance of a Birth Partner

A birth partner plays a vital role in offering comprehensive support, encompassing emotional, physical, and practical aspects, throughout the process of childbirth. This person can fulfill various roles, including being a spouse, partner, friend, family member, or a professional like a doula. Their involvement and support can significantly improve the birthing experience.

Role: Provides ongoing emotional, physical, and practical support throughout the entire labor and delivery process.

Qualities: It is important to have someone you can rely on, who comprehends your birth preferences and can speak up for you.

Emotional Support:

Providing support and reassurance can help to boost the laboring woman's confidence and maintain a sense of calm.

Consistent Presence: Remaining present throughout the labor process can offer significant emotional support and alleviate feelings of isolation.

Physical Support:

Methods for Comfort: Utilizing various techniques like massage, acupressure, and adjustments in positioning to effectively alleviate pain and discomfort.

Supporting the laboring woman by providing guidance and support in breathing exercises and relaxation techniques to help her stay focused and calm.

Advocacy:

Facilitating Effective Communication: Ensuring that the birthing woman's preferences, as outlined in the birth plan, are effectively communicated to healthcare providers.

Providing support for decision-making by aiding in the comprehension of medical information and facilitating informed choices during unforeseen circumstances.

Practical Assistance:

Practical Tasks: Overseeing the timing of contractions, offering refreshments, and ensuring the laboring woman's comfort.

Environmental Control: Establishing a serene atmosphere through the manipulation of lighting, the incorporation of gentle melodies, and the utilization of fragrant scents.

Deciding on the Best Healthcare Provider

Choosing the appropriate healthcare provider is crucial to ensure a positive and secure birth experience. This provider can be chosen based on your personal preferences and medical requirements, with options including obstetricians, midwives, or family doctors.

Responsibilities: Offers medical care, closely monitors the health of both the mother and baby, and effectively handles any potential complications that may arise.

Desirable qualities: Experience, support for your birth plan, and effective communication.

- **Qualifications and Experience:**

Verify the credentials of the provider by checking their license and ensuring they possess the required qualifications and certifications.

Seek out a provider who has a wealth of knowledge in assisting with births, especially those that align with your birth preferences (such as natural childbirth or VBAC).

Philosophy and Approach:

Consider selecting a provider whose birth philosophy is in line with your own, regardless of whether it leans towards a medical or natural approach.

Practices for Intervention: Gain insight into the provider's perspective on interventions such as inductions, epidurals, and cesarean sections.

- **Effective Communication:**

The provider should be willing to engage in discussions regarding your questions, concerns, and preferences.

- **Comfort Level:**

It is important to feel at ease and well-supported by the provider, establishing a strong sense of trust and rapport.

Advocating for Your Birth Plan

Respecting Preferences: The provider should demonstrate a willingness to honor and work within the guidelines of your birth plan.

Adaptability: Seek out a provider who is open to adjustments and willing to accommodate any necessary changes.

Reviewing the facility policies: It is important to verify that the hospital or birthing center you choose has policies that are in line with your birth plan and personal preferences.

Support Services: Ensure that support services such as lactation consultants, doulas, and postpartum care are readily available.

Creating a Supportive Birth Team: A supportive birth team is made up of individuals who play a crucial role in fostering a positive and empowering birth experience. This team may consist of healthcare providers, a birth partner, a doula, and other individuals providing support.

Doula:

Role: A highly skilled individual who offers non-medical assistance, encompassing emotional support, physical comfort, and informative guidance.

Desirable qualities: Prior experience, a composed disposition, and a steadfast dedication to upholding your birth preferences.

Family and Friends:

Role: Offers comprehensive assistance and support throughout the entire process of pregnancy, childbirth, and postpartum.

Characteristics: It is important for them to be understanding of your birth preferences and provide encouragement without causing additional pressure.

Expert in lactation:

Role: Offers expert assistance for breastfeeding, ensuring a smooth and successful beginning.

Desirable attributes for a candidate include having the necessary certifications, a wealth of experience, and a supportive nature.

Steps to Building Your Birth Team

➢ Clarify Your Needs and Preferences:

Assess the type of assistance required and envision your desired birth encounter. This assists in determining the individuals who would be best suited for your team.

➢ Conducting research and interviews:

Conduct a thorough investigation of potential team members, which may include healthcare providers and doulas. Conduct interviews to identify individuals who share your values and preferences.

➢ Share Your Birth Plan:

Make sure to communicate your birth plan to every team member so that they have a clear understanding and can provide the necessary support. Consistently assess and revise the plan as necessary.

➢ Clarify and define the various roles and responsibilities:

It is important to establish clear roles and responsibilities for each team member in order to facilitate seamless coordination and provide adequate support during the labor and delivery process.

➢ Develop a Connection:

Invest time in cultivating relationships with your birth team members to cultivate trust and open lines of communication. Make it a point to attend prenatal visits, meetings, and classes together whenever you can.

Through a meticulous process of selecting and assembling a birth team, you have the ability to cultivate an environment that fosters positivity and empowerment during your childbirth journey. Every team member plays a vital role in assisting you in achieving a birth that is free from pain and filled with joy.

CHAPTER FIVE

Methods for Alleviating Pain Naturally

Acupuncture and acupressure are both alternative therapies that have been used for centuries. They involve the application of pressure or the insertion of thin needles into specific points on the body to promote healing and relieve pain. These practices have gained popularity in recent years as people seek out natural and holistic approaches to healthcare.

Acupuncture:

Acupuncture is a practice that entails the careful insertion of thin, sterile needles into specific points on the body referred to as acupoints. These points are associated with pathways or meridians that facilitate the flow of energy, or "qi."

An expert acupuncturist skillfully identifies acupoints associated with labor pain and relaxation. Inserting needles into these points helps activate the body's natural pain-relief mechanisms. The needles can remain in position for approximately 20-30 minutes as the patient takes a moment to unwind.

Advantages:

- Diminishes labor pain by stimulating the release of endorphins.
- Promotes a sense of calmness and alleviates stress.
- May assist in stimulating labor and maintaining regular contractions.

Acupressure:

Acupressure entails the application of pressure to the acupoints utilized in acupuncture, minus the need for needles. Pressure is exerted using fingers, thumbs, or specialized tools. Continue using this technique as necessary throughout labor to effectively cope with pain and discomfort.

Advantages:

- Offers a pain relief solution that is non-invasive and user-friendly.
- Can be utilized by the birthing woman or a partner, providing instant and uninterrupted relief.
- Encourages a sense of calm and helps alleviate tension.

Massage and Aromatherapy

Massage and aromatherapy are effective therapies that can greatly alleviate labor pain and enhance the birthing experience.

Massage is a practice that involves skillfully manipulating the soft tissues of the body to alleviate pain and tension.

Massage Techniques for Labor:

- Effleurage: Gentle, circular stroking movements on the abdomen, back, or thighs to promote a sense of calm and relaxation.
- Counter-Pressure: Applying firm pressure to the lower back or hips to alleviate discomfort during contractions.
- Kneading: Deep pressure is applied to muscle groups in order to alleviate tension and enhance circulation.

Advantages:

- Alleviates muscle tension and discomfort.
- Promotes a sense of calm and helps alleviate stress.
- Promotes the activation of endorphins, the body's innate pain relievers.

Exploring the World of Aromatherapy

Aromatherapy harnesses the power of essential oils derived from plants to enhance both physical and emotional well-being.

Essential oils can be diffused in the air, incorporated into a bath, or blended with a carrier oil for massage purposes. The inhalation of these oils has the ability to stimulate the olfactory system, leading to potential effects on brain chemistry that may induce a state of relaxation.

Essential Oils for Labor:

Lavender: Known for its calming and soothing properties, it aids in reducing anxiety and promoting relaxation.

Peppermint: Stimulating and energizing, may aid in relieving nausea and enhancing vitality.

Clary Sage: Recognized for its potential to alleviate labor discomfort and stimulate uterine contractions.

Advantages:

- Promotes a sense of calmness and alleviates feelings of unease.
- Offers a delightful sensory encounter.
- Can assist in the management of pain and discomfort using natural methods.

Chiropractic Care

Chiropractic care is centered around the diagnosis and treatment of musculoskeletal problems, with a particular emphasis on the spine. This is achieved through the use of manual adjustments and various other techniques. Chiropractic care during pregnancy focuses on gentle adjustments and manipulations to address spinal misalignments, enhance pelvic alignment, and relieve nerve pressure.

Chiropractors employ specialized techniques designed for pregnant women to prioritize safety and maximize effectiveness.

How it Functions:

Spinal Adjustments: Enhancing the alignment of the spine to optimize nervous system function and enhance overall body mechanics.

Pelvic Adjustments: Ensuring the pelvis is correctly aligned to maximize comfort during labor and create an ideal environment for the baby.

Soft Tissue Therapy: Utilizing various techniques such as massage, stretching, and myofascial release to address muscle tension and enhance circulation.

Advantages:

- Relieves discomfort: Alleviates back pain, pelvic pain, and sciatica often encountered during pregnancy.
- Enhanced Pelvic Alignment: Enhances pelvic positioning for labor and delivery, potentially minimizing the duration and intensity of labor.
- Improved Nervous System Function: Enhances overall health and well-being through the enhancement of communication within the nervous system.
- Relief from Pregnancy Discomforts: Eases common discomforts like headaches, joint pain, and muscle stiffness.

Important Factors to Keep in Mind:

It is crucial to find a chiropractor with ample experience and specialized training in prenatal care. Make sure the chiropractor utilizes methods that are tailored for pregnancy. It is important to seek guidance from your healthcare provider before beginning any new treatment, as regular chiropractic care can provide benefits during pregnancy.

By integrating acupuncture, acupressure, massage, aromatherapy, and chiropractic care into your pregnancy and labor plan, you can develop a holistic and natural approach to pain relief and overall well-being. Every method provides distinct advantages and can be customized to suit your individual requirements and preferences, enhancing the overall comfort and positivity of the childbirth process.

Strategies for a Pain-Free Birth

Early Labor: Remaining Calm and Comfortable

Early labor, also known as the latent period, marks the start of the labor process. Contractions begin, but are usually moderate and irregular. This phase can continue several hours or even days. Keeping calm and comfortable is essential throughout this period.

Recognizing early labor:

- Signs include mild to moderate contractions lasting 5-30 minutes.

- Lower back ache or cramping, akin to menstruation cramps.

- There is a possibility of losing the mucus plug and seeing mild spotting.

- This phase might range from a few hours to several days.

Staying Calm:

- Deep breathing exercises might help maintain a peaceful state.

- Inhale deeply through the nose, then slowly exhale through the mouth.

- Use guided imagery to envision a peaceful and happy birth experience.

- Imagine a serene environment or a smooth labor procedure.

- Relaxing music or nature noises might help with aromatherapy.

- To induce relaxation, try using essential oils such as lavender or chamomile.

-

Staying Comfortable:

- To maximize energy for labor, prioritize relaxation and sleep.

- To be more comfortable, lie on your side with a pillow between your knees.

- Maintain proper hydration and nutrition by consuming water, herbal tea, or clear drinks.

- Eat light, easy-to-digest snacks like fruits, yogurt, or crackers.

- Warm baths or showers can relax muscles and ease tension.

- Short walks can aid in labor progression and alleviate discomfort.

- Try mild stretching or prenatal yoga.

Active Labor: Moving and Positioning.

Active labor is distinguished by stronger, more regular contractions that occur closer together. This period necessitates increased focus and energy. Movement and positioning can aid with pain management and labor progression.

Recognizing Active Labor:

- Symptoms include strong, consistent contractions every 3-5 minutes lasting 45-60 seconds.

- Increased pain and discomfort.

- Cervical dilatation ranges from 4 to 7 centimeters.

- Typically, 4-8 hours but can vary.

Moving and positioning:

- Walking and swaying can assist labor proceed and lessen pain.

- To reduce discomfort during contractions, sway your hips side to side.

- Sit on a birthing ball and gently bounce or rock to reduce pressure on your lower back.

- Use the ball to support squatting or leaning positions.

- To relieve back pressure, lean forward on a chair, bed, or partner while kneeling.

- Kneel on all fours or employ a hands-and-knees position to aid in back labor.

- Use a supported squat to expand the pelvis and move the baby down.

- Hold on to a companion or a solid piece of furniture for support.

- Rest and relax by lying on your side with a pillow between your legs.

- This position might also aid to slow down a fast labor.

To relieve pain and soothe muscles during labor, consider using a warm bath or birthing pool.

Transition and Delivery: Focus and Push

The transition period is the most intense part of labor, culminating in complete dilatation. The baby is then delivered by being pushed out. During this period, it is critical to focus and use effective pushing techniques.

Recognizing Transitions:

- Signs include severe contractions every 2-3 minutes lasting 60-90 seconds.

- Increased pressure in the lower back and rectum.

- Cervical dilatation ranges from 8 to 10 cm.

- Typically, between 30 minutes and 2 hours.

Focusing During Transition:

- Use rhythmic breathing to focus and manage pain.

- Use breathing strategies such as slow, deep breaths or short, rapid breaths as needed.

- Continue using visualization techniques to maintain a good mindset.

- Imagine the baby going down the delivery canal with each contraction.

- Seek reassurance and encouragement from your birth partner and support team.

- To maintain focus, utilize vocal affirmations and a soft touch.

Effective Pushing during Delivery:

- Push instinctively during contractions.

- Push only when you feel the need, rather than on a defined schedule.

Positions for Pushing:

- Squatting, standing, or using a birthing stool can allow gravity to assist with delivery.

- Hands and Knees: This position can help reduce back pain and open the pelvis.

- Side-lying: Provides rest and allows you greater control over the rate of pressing.

Breathing techniques:

- Take a deep breath and press down with each contraction.

- Exhale softly while pressing to keep your focus and control.

- Follow your healthcare provider's guidance to push successfully.

- Concentrate on long, prolonged pushes rather than short, strong ones.

You can improve your childbirth experience by remaining calm and comfortable during early labor, moving and employing effective positions during active labor, and focusing and applying effective pushing techniques during transition and delivery. Each stage of labor necessitates a distinct strategy for managing pain and facilitating progress, and knowing these approaches will help you navigate the process with confidence and ease.

CHAPTER SIX

Medical Pain Relief Options

Medical pain relief options can greatly alleviate or eliminate pain during childbirth. Gaining a comprehensive understanding of these options, their mechanisms, and the potential advantages and drawbacks can empower you to make well-informed decisions regarding your labor and delivery experience.

➢ **Epidural Anesthesia:**

A regional anesthesia that effectively numbs the lower part of the body, providing relief from pain.

A catheter is carefully inserted into the epidural space of the spine. A numbing drug is administered through the catheter, providing relief to the lower body.

Advantages:

- Offers substantial pain relief or complete numbness from the waist down.

- Enables you to stay awake and attentive throughout the process of labor and delivery.

Factors to Keep in Mind:

- May potentially lead to a decrease in blood pressure.

- May impede the progress of labor and potentially necessitate interventions like forceps or vacuum delivery.

- Possible side effects may manifest as itching, shivering, or challenges with urination.

➢ **Spinal Block:**

SB is an anesthetic Administered through a single injection into the spinal fluid, which offers temporary pain relief. The anesthetic is injected it into the spinal fluid in the lower back. The relief from pain is immediate and typically lasts for approximately 1-2 hours.

Advantages:

- Offers fast and efficient pain relief.

- Commonly utilized for cesarean sections or in the advanced stages of labor.

- Potential hazards and factors to take into account:

- Comparable to an epidural, but providing a briefer period of pain relief.

- Possible occurrence of a decrease in blood pressure and additional accompanying effects.

➢ **Combined Spinal-Epidural (CSE) procedure:**

It Blends in the advantages of a spinal block and an epidural. A spinal injection offers instant pain relief. A catheter is inserted to provide ongoing pain management.

Advantages:

- Instantaneous relief from the spinal block.

- Consistent pain management provided by the epidural.

Potential hazards and factors to take into account:

- Comparable to the effects of epidural and spinal block.

- There is a heightened potential for adverse effects when both techniques are used together.

> **Nitrous Oxide:**

A gas that is inhaled through a mask or mouthpiece to offer pain relief and induce relaxation. You breathe in the gas during contractions to alleviate discomfort and promote relaxation. The gas has a rapid onset and its effects diminish swiftly once inhalation ceases.

Advantages:

- Offers a moderate level of pain relief and promotes relaxation.

- Empowering individuals to have full autonomy and authority over their own usage.

Potential Side Effects:

- Possible symptoms include dizziness, nausea, or a feeling of disconnection.

- Not as potent for intense pain when compared to alternative approaches.

➢ **Opioid Analgesics:**

Medications like morphine, fentanyl, or stadol are administered through injection or IV to alleviate pain. Relief from pain is experienced within minutes and can provide several hours of comfort.

Advantages:

- Offers a moderate level of pain relief.

- Can be utilized during the initial stages of labor or in cases where an epidural is not preferred.

Potential hazards and factors to take into account:

- May result in feelings of drowsiness, nausea, or vomiting.

- May impact the newborn's respiration and level of consciousness upon delivery.

Making Educated Decisions

When it comes to making decisions about pain relief during childbirth, it's important to be well-informed. Take the time to explore your options, take into account your personal preferences and circumstances, and have an open discussion with your healthcare provider.

1. Expand Your Knowledge:

Explore various pain relief options, including both medical and natural alternatives.

Gain a comprehensive understanding of the advantages, drawbacks, and possible adverse outcomes associated with each alternative.

2. Evaluate Your Preferences:

Take into account your ability to withstand pain and your personal choices for pain management.

Consider your birth plan and how pain relief aligns with your overall vision for childbirth.

3. **Engage in a conversation with your healthcare provider:**

Engage in a thoughtful discussion with your doctor or midwife regarding the various choices available for pain relief.

Feel free to inquire and voice any apprehensions you may have regarding the various approaches.

4. **Take into account your health and work situation:**

The suitability of different pain relief options can be influenced by factors such as your health, any pregnancy complications, and the progress of your labor.

Remain adaptable and receptive to adjusting your plan if needed.

5. Develop a Birth Plan:

Consider incorporating your choices for pain relief into your birth plan.

Discuss your birth plan with your healthcare provider and birth team.

Blending Natural and Medical Approaches

Combining natural and medical methods for pain relief can offer a well-rounded and adaptable approach to coping with labor pain.

➤ **Exploring Different Approaches:**

Explore alternative pain relief techniques like breathing exercises, massage, and hydrotherapy to help manage discomfort during the early stages of labor.

If labor becomes more intense or if you feel the need for additional pain management, it may be appropriate to consider transitioning to medical pain relief options.

➢ **Customized Pain Management:**

Customize your pain relief plan to suit your unique needs and the progress of your labor.

Embrace a variety of approaches to optimize your comfort and enhance your overall experience.

➢ **Encouraging Birth Team:**

Make sure your birth team is well-informed about both natural and medical pain relief options.

Ensure that you effectively convey your preferences and any modifications to your pain relief plan to your team.

> **Adaptability and a willingness to embrace new ideas:**

Stay open-minded and ready to adjust your pain relief strategy as labor unfolds.

Recognize that it is perfectly acceptable to alter your perspective on pain relief choices as your needs and circumstances develop.

Postpartum Considerations:

Take into account the potential impact of different pain relief options on your postpartum recovery.

Consider developing a comprehensive plan for providing extra assistance and attention, tailored to the specific method of pain management employed during childbirth.

Through a thorough understanding of medical pain relief options, making well-informed choices, and incorporating both natural and medical approaches, you have the ability to develop a comprehensive pain management plan that is in line with your preferences and requirements. This will result in a childbirth experience that is more positive and empowering.

CHAPTER SEVEN

Postpartum Care: Healing and Recovery After Birth

Following childbirth, the body undergoes a substantial healing process. Gaining knowledge about what lies ahead and how to provide the necessary support can contribute to a seamless transition into the postpartum phase.

> **Mental Rehabilitation:**

Postpartum contractions aid in the natural process of the uterus returning to its pre-pregnancy size. These sensations can be experienced more profoundly during breastfeeding as a result of the release of oxytocin.

Postpartum Bleeding: Anticipate the presence of lochia, a natural discharge consisting of blood, mucus, and uterine tissue, which typically persists for a few weeks.

Perineal Care: Following vaginal births, it is common for the perineum to experience swelling or discomfort, particularly in cases where tears or an episiotomy occurred. Utilize ice packs, sitz baths, and pain relievers as necessary.

Cesarean Recovery: For those who underwent a C-section, it is important to properly care for the incision site by ensuring it remains clean and dry. Be vigilant for indications of infection, such as the presence of redness, swelling, or any abnormal discharge.

➤ **Rest and Nutrition:**

Rest: Make sure to prioritize rest and sleep when the baby sleeps in order to support your body's healing and recovery process.

Nutrition: Consume a well-rounded diet that includes ample protein, fiber, and nourishing fats. It is important to maintain proper hydration to promote breastfeeding and aid in your overall recovery.

➢ **Pelvic Floor Health:**

Enhance your pelvic floor muscles with Kegel exercises to promote bladder control and pelvic health.

Physical Therapy: It may be worth considering a visit to a pelvic floor physical therapist if you are dealing with ongoing problems like incontinence or pelvic pain.

➢ **Nursing:**

Latching and Positioning: Effective latching and positioning are crucial for preventing nipple soreness and ensuring a healthy milk supply.

Proper Hydration and Diet: Ensure adequate fluid intake and consume a nourishing diet to promote milk production.

Dealing with Postpartum Pain and Discomfort

Postpartum pain and discomfort are frequently experienced, but there are numerous methods to effectively manage them.

Relieving Pain:

Over-the-Counter Pain Relievers: Medications such as ibuprofen or acetaminophen are effective in managing pain and reducing inflammation.

Prescription Medications: In cases of intense pain, your healthcare provider may recommend more potent pain relievers.

Discomfort in the Perineal Area:

Ice Packs: Use ice packs on the perineal area to decrease swelling and alleviate discomfort.

Take a sitz bath by immersing yourself in warm water to provide relief to the perineal area and aid in the healing process.

Hemorrhoids:

Topical Treatments: Utilize readily available creams or wipes with witch hazel to alleviate discomfort and inflammation.

Optimize your diet by incorporating foods rich in fiber and staying hydrated to promote regularity and minimize discomfort when passing stools.

Dealing with Breast Engorgement and Nipple Pain:

Applying warm compresses to the breasts before breastfeeding can be beneficial in facilitating milk flow.

Utilize cold compresses in between feedings to alleviate any discomfort and reduce swelling.

Use lanolin or other nipple creams to provide relief and promote healing for cracked or sore nipples.

Pain from Cesarean Section:

Incision Care: It is important to maintain cleanliness and dryness at the site of the incision, while also adhering to the care instructions provided by your healthcare provider.

Activity: Engaging in gentle movement and walking can support the healing process and reduce the risk of blood clots.

Emotional well-being and mental health

The postpartum period can be mentally demanding. Recognizing the significance of your psychological well-being is equally crucial to your physical recuperation.

Postpartum Emotions:

Baby Blues: It's normal to go through mood swings, bouts of crying, and feelings of anxiety during the initial two weeks after giving birth as a result of hormonal fluctuations.

Postpartum Depression: If feelings of sadness, hopelessness, or anxiety continue for more than two weeks, it is possible that you are experiencing postpartum depression. Consult a healthcare professional for assistance.

Systems of Support:

Partner and Family Support: Rely on your loved ones for both emotional and practical assistance.

Support Groups: Connect with other new mothers by joining postpartum support groups. They can provide a valuable understanding of your experiences.

Mindful Practices:

Make sure to set aside some time for activities that bring you joy and help you unwind, like reading a good book, going for a leisurely walk, or indulging in a soothing bath.

Embrace the power of mindfulness and meditation to effectively handle stress and enhance your emotional well-being.

Expert Assistance:

Therapy: It may be beneficial to consult with a therapist or counselor who has expertise in postpartum concerns.

Medical Professional: Regular appointments with your healthcare provider can assist in monitoring your emotional and physical recovery.

Striking a harmonious equilibrium Duties:

Seek Assistance: Feel free to seek assistance with household tasks, childcare, or other responsibilities without any hesitation.

Establish Reasonable Anticipations: Recognize that the process of recovery requires patience and it is perfectly acceptable to proceed at a leisurely pace.

By emphasizing the importance of healing and recovery, addressing postpartum pain and discomfort, and prioritizing emotional well-being and mental health, you can help facilitate a smoother transition into motherhood and promote a healthy and positive postpartum experience.

Bonding with Your Baby

The Significance of Skin-to-Skin Contact

Placing your newborn on your bare chest, skin to skin, is a practice known as kangaroo care. This practice provides a multitude of advantages for both the baby and the parents.

Benefits for the Baby's Physical Well-being:

Temperature Regulation: Skin-to-skin contact aids in maintaining the baby's body temperature, ensuring their warmth and comfort.

Direct contact has a stabilizing effect on the newborn's heart rate and breathing patterns.

Enhanced Weight Gain: Encourages healthier eating patterns and can result in enhanced weight gain.

Decreased Stress: Reduces levels of stress hormones in the baby, promoting a sense of calm and security.

Benefits for the Mind and Emotions:

Strengthening the emotional bond between the baby and the parents, fostering a sense of security and attachment.

Babies held skin-to-skin experience a decrease in crying and are more easily comforted.

Improved Brain Development: Supports the growth and function of the brain by providing sensory stimulation and fostering bonding.

Advantages for Parents:

Fosters Connection: Facilitates a profound emotional bond with the newborn.

Enhances Breast Milk Production: The close proximity of the baby triggers the release of hormones that stimulate an increase in breast milk production.

Enhances Confidence: Assists parents in developing a stronger sense of assurance and connection in their role, alleviating worry and fostering a feeling of overall wellness.

Methods for Engaging in Skin-to-Skin Contact:

Begin promptly after birth and maintain regularity during the initial weeks.

Optimal Position: Embrace the baby gently against your warm chest, providing a cozy environment by draping a blanket over both of you. Ensure the baby's head is gently turned to the side for added comfort.

Both parents: Promote the involvement of both parents in skin-to-skin time to enhance the development of a strong bond.

Fundamentals and Advantages of Breastfeeding

Breastfeeding is known to provide the best nutrition for your baby and has been found to have numerous health benefits for both the baby and the mother.

Breast milk provides a well-rounded combination of nutrients, antibodies, and hormones that are crucial for the baby's growth and development. Breast milk is more easily digested by babies in comparison to formula.

Benefits for the Baby's Health:

Enhancing Immunity: Offers antibodies that aid in safeguarding the baby against infections and illnesses.

Decreased Risk of Chronic Conditions: Decreases the risk of various conditions including asthma, obesity, diabetes, and Sudden Infant Death Syndrome (SIDS).

Advantages for the Mother

Facilitates Bonding: Breastfeeding facilitates a strong emotional bond between mother and baby.

Health Benefits: Decreases the likelihood of experiencing postpartum depression and lowers the risk of developing specific forms of cancer (breast and ovarian cancer). Additionally, it aids in the restoration of the uterus to its original size before pregnancy.

Efficient Calorie Burning: Facilitates the burning of additional calories and aids in achieving postpartum weight loss.

Breastfeeding Techniques:

Proper Latching: It is important to ensure that the baby has a deep latch, with the mouth covering most of the areola, rather than just the nipple.

Try out various breastfeeding positions (such as cradle, cross-cradle, football hold, side-lying) to determine the most effective one for you and your baby.

Observing Feeding Cues: It is beneficial to observe early feeding cues like rooting, sucking on hands, or smacking lips, instead of waiting for the baby to cry.

Typical Obstacles and Resolutions:

For relief from sore nipples, try using lanolin cream or expressed breast milk.

For optimal results, it is recommended to use warm compresses before feeding and cold compresses afterward to help alleviate swelling.

Insufficient Milk Production: Consider increasing the frequency of feedings, ensuring a proper latch, and seeking guidance from a lactation specialist if necessary.

➤ **Developing a Solid Parent-Child Bond**

Developing a solid parent-child bond establishes the groundwork for a positive, stable, and affectionate relationship.

Analyzing Responsive Parenting:

Be attentive and responsive to your baby's cries and cues, as this helps to build trust and a sense of security.

Regularly holding, cuddling, and comforting your baby can help strengthen the emotional bond between you and your little one.

Communication:

Engage in verbal communication by talking, singing, and reading to your baby, even from birth. This supports the growth of language skills and fosters a strong emotional connection.

Eye Contact: Sustaining eye contact during feedings and interactions can strengthen the bond and facilitate effective communication.

Establishing a regular routine and maintaining consistency:

Developing consistent routines for feeding, sleeping, and playtime can help provide a sense of security and predictability for your baby.

Create unique routines, like sharing bedtime stories or enjoying morning cuddles, to enhance the connection between you and your loved ones.

Play and Interaction:

Engage in play activities that are suitable for your baby's age and help stimulate their senses while promoting the development of cognitive and motor skills.

Engage in interactive play by using toys, mirrors, and fun games like peek-a-boo to foster joy and encourage participation.

Taking care of oneself as a parent:

Make your mental and emotional well-being a top priority. A parent's well-being significantly impacts their ability to form strong bonds and provide proper care for their child.

Request Assistance: Seek assistance from loved ones, close friends, or support groups to effectively navigate the complexities of parenting.

By emphasizing skin-to-skin contact, promoting breastfeeding, and cultivating a strong parent-child bond, you can establish a caring and encouraging atmosphere that nurtures your baby's physical, emotional, and cognitive growth, while also enriching your own parenting journey.

CHAPTER EIGHT

An Introspective Look at Your Birth Experience

One of the most powerful and healing processes you can go through is to take some time to reflect on your birth journey. It gives you the opportunity to reflect on your experiences, acknowledge your accomplishments, and gain wisdom from any difficulties you had.

Recognizing the Value of Your Experience:

Take some time to reflect on your birth experience by writing in a notebook or having a conversation with someone about it. Recognize the feelings that you experienced as well as the accomplishments that you gained.

Sharing Your Story: If you are interested in sharing your birth story with others, you might want to think about doing so through a support group, social media, or a blog. Other people who are expecting can find support and inspiration from your tale.

Gaining Knowledge and Developing Oneself:

The process of identifying strengths involves acknowledging the qualities and resiliency that you displayed throughout the labor and delivery process. Your ability to remain calm, focused, and empowered is something you should reflect on.

Taking on Challenges: Take some time to think about any difficulties or unforeseen occurrences that have taken place. Think about the things you've picked up from these encounters and how they might impact the choices you make in the future or the advice you give to other people.

Recognizing and Honoring Successes:

Celebrate all of the significant and insignificant milestones that you have attained, from the beginning of your labor through the contractions to the time that you gave birth.

Cherish the early moments of bonding with your newborn and the special journey you went on together. These are the moments that you will remember forever.

Inspiring and enabling future generations

Your experiences and the knowledge you've obtained can serve as a source of inspiration for parents of the next generation. The act of sharing your observations and experiences contributes to the formation of a community that is supportive and in which new parents feel knowledgeable and confident.

As you come to the end of this phase of your life, remember to carry with you the knowledge, the fortitude, and the empowerment that you have acquired. Listed below are some concluding ideas and words of inspiration to keep moving forward.

Give Yourself Trust:

Have faith in the strength and wisdom that are within you. In spite of the fact that you went through one of the most significant events of your life, you have emerged more powerful and knowledgeable. Always put your faith in your gut feelings when it comes to parenting. You have a deeper understanding of both yourself and your child than anybody else.

Seek Out Assistance:

Being a parent is a never-ending process of acquiring new knowledge. Make sure you don't be afraid to seek assistance, inquire about things, and make connections with people who may provide direction. Surround yourself with a group that is encouraging and supportive with the goal of elevating and encouraging you. When you find yourself in need, lean on your support system.

Accept and Embrace the Trip:

Be patient and kind with yourself as you negotiate the ups and downs of parenthood. Maintain a sympathetic and caring attitude toward yourself. There is no shame in making errors and gaining knowledge along the way. Embrace the moments of delight and show gratitude for the modest victories and beautiful moments you have with your child.

Foster the Empowerment of Others:

The trip you have taken has the potential to inspire others. Your experience should be shared, you should offer your support, and you should be a source of inspiration for people who are beginning their own journeys toward becoming parents.

Looking to the Future:

Possibilities for the Future: It is important to have a positive and enthusiastic outlook on the future. Every stage of parenting brings with it a new set of experiences and chances for personal development.

Leaving a Legacy of Love: Leave behind a legacy of love, support, and empowerment that will have a beneficial impact not just on your child but also on future generations.

It is important to keep in mind that you are not alone as you go forward. You are a member of a bigger community of parents who are all working toward the same goal of becoming the greatest possible parents for themselves and their children. The road you have taken should be celebrated, the future should be welcomed, and you should continue to empower others by sharing the knowledge and strength you have learned.

Hospital Bag Checklist for Labor and Delivery

Mother's Essentials

ID Card and Insurance Information: Required for hospital admission and processing.

Birth Plan: Please share a copy of your birth plan with the medical staff.

Hospital Registration Forms: If you pre-registered, please bring any required documentation.

Comfort and Clothing:

Robe and nightgown: Comfortable and simple to open for breastfeeding and examination.

Slippers and Socks: Warm socks and non-slip slippers for added comfort and safety.

Comfortable Outfits: Dress loosely and comfortably for your hospital stay and return travel.

Nursing bras and pads make breastfeeding more comfortable and convenient.

Underwear: High-waisted, comfy underwear, preferably disposable or ones you don't mind getting dirty.

Toiletries & Personal Care:

Toothbrush with toothpaste.

Hairbrush and Ties

Lip Balm: Hospitals can be dry.

Moisturizer and facial wipes: To refresh and stay moisturized.

Shampoo, Conditioner, Body Wash: Travel-sized for convenience.

Deodorant and Labor Comfort Items:

Massage Oil or Lotion: Provides comfort during labor.

If the hospital allows it, use a birth ball to aid with labor progression and comfort.

Pillows: Use your own pillow for comfort.

Music or relaxation? Aids include a playlist, headphones, and portable speakers.

Essential Oils: If you find aromatherapy beneficial.

Food and Drink:

Snacks and Drinks: Easy-to-eat snacks such as granola bars, almonds, and electrolyte drinks can provide energy throughout and after labor.

Entertainment and distractions:

To pass the time during early labor, read books, magazines, or use a tablet.

Phone and charger: For staying in touch with family and friends.

Essential items for the partner or support person include comfortable clothing and toiletries.

Change of Clothes:

Dress comfortably during your hospital stay.

Toiletries include toothbrushes, toothpaste, deodorant, and other basics.

Pillow and Blanket: For resting during lengthy labor hours.

Essential Baby Clothing and Accessories:

Onesies and sleepers: Several infant clothes, including one for going home.

Socks and mittens: These will keep the infant warm and avoid scratching.

Hats provide warmth, especially in cooler temperatures.

Receiving Blankets and Swaddles Blankets: For swaddling and keeping warm.

Diapers and wipes:

Newborn Diapers: Although the hospital normally gives these, it's a good idea to have some on hand.

Baby Wipes are sensitive, unscented wipes for infant skin.

Food Supplies:

Formula and Bottles: If you intend to bottle-feed.

Breastfeeding Pillow: Makes nursing more pleasant.

Car Seats:

Infant Car Seat: Securely placed in your vehicle for the drive home.

Packing these necessities ensures that you have all you need for a comfortable and prepared hospital stay throughout labor and delivery.

END